Yoga 101:

Simple Yoga Poses to Calm Your Mind & Energize Your Body

Max Fischwell

ISBN-13: 978-1499709445

ISBN-10: 1499709447

About the Author

Max Fischwell is about improving his life in various ways, and loves to share what he has accomplished by writing books so that his readers can learn to improve themselves as well.

One of his favorite past-times is to stay fit both physically and mentally. Therefore, one of his favorite endeavors that he has recently embarked upon is practicing yoga and meditation.

Max Fischwell loves yoga as it keeps you fit physically as well as mentally. However since meditation is an important aspect of yoga, Max Fischwell has taken a profound interest in studying meditation and loves practicing it, as it also has great benefits mentally by itself.

Right now Max Fischwell is in the process of maintaining his health from cardio and yoga and is always looking for ways he can educate and improve himself.

Table of Contents

Max Fischwell

Word of Caution:

If you are pregnant or have any physical ailments please consult a doctor or professional before you proceed with Yoga. While yoga is usually safe and sometimes even recommended, it is essential to consult a professional to make sure it is safe, and if there are any limitations or adjustments that need to be made due to your condition.

Why Practice Yoga?

Although the Eastern practice of yoga was first developed in India
thousands of years ago, it has recently gained tremendous popularity in
the West as a modern-day symbol of inner peace, tranquility, and
health. In fact, the 2012 Yoga in America study from Yoga Journal
found that 20.4 million Americans practice yoga regularly, a whopping
increase of 29 percent since 2008.

Despite the fact that research on yoga is still young, studies have
already indicated that the health benefits of the mind-body practice
rival some other popular forms of exercise, including jogging and
aerobics. So far, the following are the proven physical and mental
health benefits linked to yoga through Western scientific research
findings.

Decreased Levels of Stress and Anxiety

Through the combined stretching, controlled breathing, and relaxation
exercises associated with yoga, it is no surprise that the practice
naturally acts as a great stress or anxiety reliever. Instead of turning to

potentially harmful medications that come with a mountain of negative side effects, many yogis depend on yoga as a vital stress management tool and rightly so.

In a 2005 study at the Department of Integrative and Internal Medicine in the University of Duisburg-Essen of Germany, researchers found that women who participated in yoga classes twice a week for three months demonstrated significant improvements in scores on both the Cohen Perceived Stress Scale and the State-Trait Anxiety Inventory. Furthermore, engaging in yoga practices was linked to a dramatic decrease in the participants' salivary cortisol levels, which is the main steroid hormone activated by stress.

In the March 2009 edition of the International Journal of Gynecology and Obstetrics, researchers studied the effects of integrated yoga practices on perceived levels of stress and measured autonomic stress responses for healthy pregnant women between their 18th and 20th week of pregnancy. While the control group in the study experienced a perceived stress increase by 6.6 percent, those practicing yoga realized a decrease in perceived stress by 31.57 percent.

Researchers also discovered that the yoga group's heart rate variability was significantly reduced with the deep relaxation techniques. Since stress has a negative effect on unborn babies, this study provides evidence that pregnant women may want to consider consulting their doctor about utilizing the power of yoga to lower their stress and anxiety levels.

Relieved Depression Symptoms

Depression is a severely impairing condition that causes individuals to suffer from low moods, fatigue, insomnia, loss of self-esteem, feelings of hopelessness, and sometimes suicidal thoughts. Similarly to antidepressant medications and psychotherapy techniques, yoga practices have been associated with positively influencing the production of chemical messengers in the brain called neurotransmitters to relieve depression.

In a 2008 study from the International Journal of Yoga Therapy, researchers from the LifeForce Yoga Healing Institute discovered that all 94 participants in their yoga retreat reported decreased levels of depression on the Beck Depression Inventory (BDI) and Profile of Mood States Questionnaire (POMS). While the average score for participants before the retreat was 94, results showed that the participants had an average score of 33 by the end of the study for a statistically significant decrease.

Published in the December 2007 edition of the journal of Evidence-Based Complementary and Alternative Medicine, researchers from the

Semel Institute for Neuroscience and Human Behavior conducted a study to examine the potential for yoga to be utilized as a complementary treatment for 27 female and 10 male patients diagnosed with unipolar major depression. After participants completed 20 yoga classes, significant reductions were found in levels of depression, anger, anxiety, heart rate variability, and neurotic symptoms. In fact, 11 of the participants even achieved remission levels for their depression after the yoga intervention. Researchers concluded that yoga is an easy, cost-effective, and promising supplement treatment option for depressed patients.

One of the common symptoms related to depression is insomnia, or disturbances in sleeping patterns. According to a 2004 study in the journal of Applied Psychophysiology and Biofeedback, researchers at the Division of Sleep Medicine at Harvard Medical School found that the relaxation and meditation of yoga is an effective treatment for reducing arousal in patients with chronic insomnia.

During the eight-week study, participants maintained sleep-wake diaries while following a yoga training session with a professional instructor. Researchers found statistically significant improvements in sleep efficiency, total sleep time, total wake time, sleep onset latency, wake time after sleep onset, and sleep quality measures at the end of the intervention.

Improved Immune System Functioning

Since yoga emphasizes total relaxation of the mind and body, it also enables the body's immune system to function at a more optimal level to carry out its duties of protecting individuals from germs and illnesses. In a 2012 study conducted by the University of California at Los Angeles and published in the journal of Psychoneuroendocrinology, researchers selected 45 participants who were under the stress of caring for a loved one with dementia. After engaging in just 12 minutes of yoga daily for eight weeks, researchers found that the caregivers significantly reduced the biological mechanisms that are responsible for increasing the inflammation response from the immune system. Lower levels of inflammation throughout the body boosts the immune system to fight off a multitude of chronic and stress-related health concerns.

While it is clear that yoga has a significant impact on improving how the human immune system works, a small 2013 Norwegian study published in the international journal PLOS ONE has discovered breakthrough genetic evidence to support this claim. Within the research, ten participants underwent a week-long yoga retreat for four-hour yoga sessions with meditation, stretching, and breathing exercises.

At the conclusion of the study, researchers examined the participants'
blood and found 111 genes changed in their expression in circulating
immune cells. In comparison, relaxation exercises through music and
walking only alter the expression of 38 genes. Therefore, the research
suggests that there is an integral physiological component at the
molecular level that causes yoga to immediately boost the immune
system.

Increased Physical Fitness

Unlike other strenuous and high-impact aerobic exercises that come
with serious disadvantages for the body, yoga is an isometric weight-
bearing exercise that has been shown to improve bone strength without
damaging cartilage. Yoga helps to stretch the muscles, increase the
individual's range of motion, and even prevent bone loss associated
with osteoporosis.

In a March 2009 study by Dr. Loren Fishman, elderly participants
were able to add more than three-fourths of a point on the DEXA bone
density tests for the spine and four-fifths of a point for the prone hip
bone with just ten short minutes of yoga practice each day. In fact,
several of the participants who had been diagnosed with osteoporosis
improved the strength of their bones enough to be re-classified with
the less severe counterpart of osteopenia.

Although the other study provided evidence of yoga improving the physical fitness level of older adults, the same is found to be true for healthy young adults. In a March 2013 longitudinal controlled investigation from the Department of Health and Exercise Science at Colorado State University, researchers found that the effects of yoga on general physical fitness span across the entire age spectrum. The young, healthy yoga subjects exhibited increased flexibility in the back, hamstrings, and shoulders. Participants also experienced enhanced deadlift strength and reduced body fat compared to the control group.

Within the July/August edition of Alternative Therapies in Health and Medicine, scientists at the Fred Hutchinson Cancer Research Center also found evidence that regular yoga practice is effective at promoting weight loss in those who are overweight, as well as preventing weight gain in middle-aged individuals who are of normal weight. In the immense study involving 15,500 participants, researchers found that men and women who practiced yoga regularly gained three fewer pounds in a ten-year frame than those who did not.

They also struck gold by discovering that overweight men and women lost about five pounds in the ten-year period while those that did not practice yoga gained 14 pounds on average. In addition to its fat-burning potential, yoga increases also physical awareness and makes individuals more sensitive to feelings of satiation to curb overeating.

Enhanced Cognition and Brain Function

It has become obvious that yoga is great for the human body, but could the practice actually help the brain function more efficiently too? Well, a recent study at the University of Illinois in the Journal of Physical Activity found that a single 20-minute session of Hatha yoga was able to significantly improve participants' performance on the Flanker Task for working memory and the N-back Task for attention span. Test scores following the short stint of yoga were significantly higher and reaction times were also considerably shorter. Interestingly enough, the control group that participated in jogging on a treadmill exhibited no increase in cognitive performance from the baseline testing.

In the December 2012 edition of the Journal of Alternative and Complementary Medicine, researchers discovered that yoga also has a strong effect on the cognitive performance of young children as well. At the start of the study and after three months of yoga intervention, the Wechsler Intelligence Scale for Children was administered to 200 schoolchildren between the ages of seven and nine. Significant improvements were realized in the cognitive functions of attention, concentration, visual-spatial abilities, verbal capabilities, and abstract thinking skills on average. Researchers concluded that yoga was as effective as other forms of physical activity in enhancing the overall cognitive performance of school aged children and high levels of attention associated with yoga may be the key to successful academic learning.

Lowered Pain Levels from Chronic Ailments

For individuals who suffer from the crippling effects of chronic pain as the result of various ailments, yoga practices have been linked to minimizing the amount of pain and improving overall quality of life. In a 2012 study published in the Journal of Pain from the American Pain Society, researchers discovered that yoga was in particular effective for treating chronic neck pain. During the nine-week research period, the 77 patients were randomized into a lyengar yoga program with weekly 90-minute classes or a self-exercise program.

Participants in the yoga group experienced an average decrease on the Visual Analog Scale (VAS) from 44.3 at baseline to 13.0 at week ten from yoga alone. Pain at motion was also reduced for the yoga participants from 53.4 to 22.4 within the nine weeks of practice. Not only did the researchers conclude that yoga is an effective treatment for chronic neck pain, they also suggested that yoga has potential positive effects on psychological well-being and quality of life for chronic pain sufferers.

More than just for neck pain, a 2011 study published in the Annals of Internal Medicine found that yoga practices are equally effective for individuals with chronic low back pain. The researchers at the University of York tracked 313 back pain patients and assigned 156 of the participants into a three-month beginner yoga training program for 75 minutes each week.

Participants completed a thorough questionnaire about their back pain levels at three months, six months, and 12 months. At the end, patients in the yoga group reported a higher decrease in pain and indicated ability to do 30 percent more daily activities than the control group. At the year mark, 60 percent of the yoga group reported continuing the practice and less back pain.

Improved Relationships and Sexual Functioning

Through the journey of self-exploration into meaning and mindfulness, yoga practices are beneficial for helping individuals manage their mental state for a happy and fulfilled romantic relationship with their partner. Yoga helps develop the self-awareness and presence that is necessary to be emotionally present with one's significant other in a world full of distractions to keep the bond strong.

Since practicing yoga has been linked to improved blood circulation and increased oxygen levels, it also provides the energy needed to maintain the burning fire of love. According to the book, Partner Yoga: Making Contact for Physical Emotional & Spiritual Growth, by author Cain Carroll; couples can strengthen their trust, patience, communication, intimacy, and acceptance by participating in various yoga practices together.

Since the ancient method of relaxation and exercise is clearly associated with improving the functioning of various areas of the human body, it should be no surprise that it can also serve as a natural enhancement for sexual function. In the 2009 edition of the Journal of Sexual Medicine, researchers studied 40 healthy women between the ages of 22 and 55 who reported being sexually active.

During the study, the women were assigned to a yoga program with 22 yoga poses believed to have positive impacts on the abdominal and pelvic muscle tone. At the end of the program, researchers found improvements in the women's sexual functioning scores in terms of desire, lubrication, arousal, orgasm, pain, and overall sexual satisfaction.

Enhanced Performance Across All Disciplines

Yoga is an appropriate practice that can be used to help individuals enhance their performance across a wide spectrum of disciplines. For athletes, yoga can help gain knowledge about the connection between the mind and body, improve mental focus, strengthen body awareness, and induce mental clarity that is necessary to excel in any sport. Physically, yoga helps athletes to lower their heart rate, increase the oxygen being taken into their lungs, strengthen their muscles, and improve flexibility.

Yoga can be particularly beneficial for athletes with a recent sports injury, in order to relieve muscle tension and lessen their recovery time without straining their muscles with intense exercise. Yoga provides a whole body workout that will enhance all cross-training programs as a perfect supplement to strong cardiovascular workouts.

While it makes the most sense that yoga helps improve athlete's abilities on and off their sports field, the ancient practices are also extremely advantageous in another discipline – music and the arts. Musicians and artists who engage in routine yoga practices benefit from improved concentration, focus, awareness of surroundings, and sparks of creativity.

Awakening their inner artist, yoga has a profound effect on enabling individuals to tap into their higher inspiration, refine their artist skills, and empower their creative expression, whether with paints, words, or songs. In a study from the journal of Applied Psychophysiology and Biofeedback, researchers discovered that yoga can also help to reduce performance anxiety and mood disturbances of professional musicians, as well as enhance their physical abilities at performing their instrument of choice.

Overall, scientists and experts in the field have found research evidence that substantially supports the claim that yoga provides tremendous physical, mental, emotional, social, psychological, behavioral, spiritual, musculoskeletal, and biological health benefits to the human body. Whatever your age or fitness level may be, yoga is hands down one of the best methods for staying healthy, looking great, and feeling fantastic. Although it may be difficult to get the hang of it at first, the benefits in the long-term far outweigh the initial confusion. Keep trying and you will be able to realize these exceptional benefits that have been scientifically linked to the ancient powers of yoga.

Yogi Prep

When beginner yogis first start practicing yoga, it is often a less than Zen-like experience. It is the unfortunate truth that many people decide to not try practicing yoga simply because they are overwhelmed with anxiety on how to get started.

However, having a fundamental understanding on how to prepare for the exercise can significantly ease the transition into yoga and calm the beginner jitters. Whether you have recently signed up for your first yoga class or are planning to begin practicing yoga at home for the first time, the following are some basic tips to both mentally and physically prepare yourself for yoga practice the right way.

Mental Preparation

Although yoga seems like mostly a physical form of exercise, yoga is just as much about the mind as it is the body. Through regular practice, yogis are able to achieve a calmer mind and reach inner peace for excellent overall mental health. However, you must prepare mentally for the practice of yoga because it is a lot more difficult than you might think.

First, make sure that you clear you mind of all distractions. Forget about the conversation you had at work with your boss or your list of unfinished chores at home. Prepare yourself for some mental downtime by focusing on your body movements and your breathing to achieve stillness of mind.

You should have formed a list of goals and objectives that you want to achieve from yoga practices prior to stepping foot on the mat. Do you simply want increase your physical health and well-being, or do you want to free yourself from anxiety and get in touch with your inner spirituality? The yogi exercises that you choose to participate in will vary greatly depending on your individual goals.

For instance, the popular downward-facing dog pose is perfect for reducing stiffness in your shoulders, but the upward-facing dog stretch is more beneficial for relieving tension in the spine. Ask yourself what you want to accomplish from yoga and do not be afraid to dig deep.

Before starting yoga, it is important that you learn how to listen. Not only will you have to mentally tune your listening skills to follow verbal directions from your yoga instructor, you will need to listen to your own body. Get in touch with your body to learn both your physical and mental limitations to know how far you can push without causing injury. While the person next to you in class may be able to stretch a bit further, always remember that yoga is not a competition.

Focus all of your mental energies inward on your own body without being self-conscious of your abilities. Despite the fact that you may look downright silly as a novice, remember that other students are there to get more mentally relaxed just like you and will not be judgmental. Most of all, stay positive!

Physical Preparation

As with any other form of exercise, you should start by checking with your physician to ensure you are physically fit for practicing yoga. This is especially important if you have any pre-existing medical conditions, including asthma, inner ear conditions, heart disease, high blood pressure, arthritis, and osteoporosis.

If you have never exercised before, have undergone surgery lately, or had a hip replacement, it is recommended that you make a trip to the doctor before engaging in yoga practices. Pregnant women should also consult with their obstetrician to learn about advisable yoga modifications that need to be made to protect the safety of both mother and child.

After you have been given the green light by a healthcare professional, it is important to begin gathering the necessary yoga equipment. If you have made the commitment to yoga and are fairly certain it is for you, it is generally recommended that you invest in purchasing a yoga mat, especially to provide cushioning on a hard floor surface.

If you will be participating in a yoga class and are strapped for cash, most venues have mats that you can rent for just a few dollars. While the only vital piece of equipment for yoga is the mat to create much-needed traction, you may want to consider having a blanket or yoga block on hand to provide elevation and support during certain poses.

When practicing yoga, it is essential that you dress comfortably in loose clothes that enable your body to move naturally. However, avoid baggy tops and pants that will likely slide up in even the most basic of poses. Fitted attire is the best option to avoid the distraction of constantly readjusting your clothes and the embarrassment of accidentally exposing too much skin. Although there are various kinds of yoga pants, there is no need to run out to buy a special pair since any exercise pants will do.

For women, it is suggested that you wear a well-fitted sports bra that will provide support, but not cause uncomfortable pinching or hinder your breathing. You can leave your socks and shoes behind because yoga is usually practiced barefoot, but remember to bring along a towel for when things start to get sweaty.

Furthermore, another helpful hint is to make sure you time eating around yoga to avoid practicing with a full stomach. While it is never recommended that you skip meals or fast on days that you do yoga, you should generally avoid eating for at least two hours before your class or home session.

When you eat this far in advance, it guarantees that your body will have the needed energy for yoga without the overly full feeling. That being said, it is crucial that you stay hydrated and drink some water before yoga however not too much where you may feel bloated. In addition to being prohibited in most classes, it is not advisable that you drink water during yoga because this has the tendency of circulating the flow of Prana downwards.

When your body and mind are properly prepared for yoga practices, you increase the likelihood of improving your concentration, lowering your blood pressure, reducing your levels of stress, strengthening your muscles, boosting your overall mood, calming your mind, and increasing your self-awareness for inner peace. Therefore, in order to gain the most rewarding mental and physical benefits, make sure that you remember to follow these basic tips to prepare for your next yoga session!

Yogic Breathing

The Importance of Proper Yogic Breathing

As one of the most basic involuntary human functions, breathing is such a simple and effortless action that most people take for granted its profound impact on the body, mind, and spirit. While we all know how to breathe because it happens automatically and spontaneously, experts indicate that most individuals today are actually breathing incorrectly.

Through our fast-paced modern world filled with stresses, most people breathe too quickly and less deeply than is intended for the human body. As a result, our bodies are not taking in a sufficient level of oxygen nor eliminating enough carbon dioxide, thus causing toxins to build up. Since the lungs are not being exercised properly, the unhealthy habit of shallow breathing can cause them to diminish in function and reduce the level of energy in every cell of the body. Going through life, these bad breathing practices become habitual and can lead to significant permanent health problems, unless the habits are properly reversed.

Therefore, yogis have realized the great importance of taking in an adequate supply of oxygen to revitalize the mind and body by perfecting various healthy breathing techniques. Pranayama, one of the five fundamental principles of yoga, refers to the science of breath control to promote proper breathing and keep the body in vibrant health. Within the yogic viewpoint, Pranayama aims to bring more oxygen into the blood and brain in order to direct prana, which is the vital force of energy that gives humans life.

Yoga breathing is one of the most beneficial methods for coping with stress and the resulting restricted breathing that dramatically drops the body's level of oxygen. Read on to find an in-depth guide on how you can implement proper breathing exercises in your yoga sessions and the incredible benefits that will boost your vitality.

Four Stages of Yoga Breathing

Despite the fact that respiration is commonly misunderstood as merely a single act of inhalation followed by a single exhalation, yoga breathing places an emphasis on four distinct stages that all have a specific purpose for achieving good overall health. Transitioning from the four phases of breathing involves reversing the flow of energy through the muscles of the body, as well as expansive or contractive movements within the lungs, chest, shoulders, and abdomen. Since it is crucial to have an understanding of these stages to implement proper yoga breathing, the following is a step-by-step look at the four phases to increase your awareness.

Puraka – As the name provided for the initial inhalation, Puraka is the process of taking in air in one smooth, continuous motion. Air is drawn into the lungs to fill the diaphragm and deliver the much-needed oxygen to the various cells of the body. Through certain yoga breathing exercises, individuals may pause one or multiple times in the process of inhalation, which is termed as a broken Puraka or series of Purakas.

Abhyantara Kumbhaka – After the oxygen is filled into the lungs, the Abhyantara Kumbhaka stage consists of a deliberate pause that stops the flow of air into the lungs and retains the oxygen within the diaphragm. While a novice may have difficulty keeping the pause completely motionless and need to follow elaborate instructions to achieve the purpose, this second phase is intended to curb all movement in the lungs and muscles of the body.

Rechaka – Similar to inhalation, the Rechaka stage involves a smooth and continuous exhalation of the oxygen out of the lungs at a slow pace. As the muscles naturally relax their tension, the air is expelled from the lungs and the organs return to their normal condition. Some yogis may exert muscular effort to force the air out of the lungs when in a seated position or erect standing pose with the abdominal muscles constricted.

Bahya Kumbhaka – The final phase of respiration known as Bahya Kumbhaka, or simply Kumbhaka, includes a deliberate pause after the act of inhalation as the body becomes empty of oxygen. After a short or prolonged stoppage, this phase completes the breathing cycle, terminates the pauses, and begins the next Puraka inhalation.

Proper Breathing in Yoga Techniques

When performing yoga exercises, it is essential that you master the skills of proper yoga breathing to get the most benefits out of your practices. However, at the same time, don't worry too much about the 4 phase breathing cycle mentioned above when doing the poses. While that is great to practice separately you may find it very difficult especially if you are a novice to implement when going through the yogic postures.

Instead what you want to focus on regarding yoga breathing during the poses is to simply allow your body to totally relax and completely release the buildup of tension. Since a relaxed body is primed deep breathing, it is imperative that you stay relaxed and focused as you move into each stage.

Beginner yogis often make the mistake of trying to over-control their breathing by forcing air in and out at a rate that is similar to hyperventilation. If you are straining your breathing, chances are high that you are not breathing correctly and are taking in too much oxygen. Rather than breathing rapidly, remain calm and allow your body to naturally take in the desired amount of oxygen that it is starving for.

You should always try to fill your diaphragm with air at a slow, leisurely pace. Intake a deep cleansing breath through your nostrils and then release it back out through slowly. It is important to breathe through your nose during proper yoga breathing because the nose is the body's natural defense mechanism to trap the pathogens that are seeking their way into the lungs.

Yogis also strongly believe that breathing through the nose enables your body to naturally absorb free energy from the air. However, if your nose is plugged or stuffy from the effects of a cold, it will be necessary to breathe through a combination of nose and mouth, or simply the mouth. With each intake, be sure to extend your breath to its comfortable maximum as deeply as you can before exhaling as fully as possible.

Furthermore, always remember to place your safety at the highest priority when engaging in yoga breathing or embarking on breath control exercises. If you have asthma, chronic respiratory problems, or heart disease, make sure to consult with your physician or healthcare provider before you start practicing yoga in any form.

Benefits of Healthy Yoga Breathing Habits

Deep breathing is the only means of supplying the single most vital nutrient to our bodies and the various organs that keep us alive. While we could survive for weeks without food and days without water, we would perish within minutes without a steady supply of oxygen. As the organ that requires more oxygen than any other, the brain desperately needs oxygen for efficient functioning.

If the body does not receive enough, it is common for individuals to be more physically or mentally sluggish, have more negative thoughts, and experience vision or hearing difficulties. Thus, yoga breathing is imperative for guaranteeing that the body is being delivered all of the healthy nutrients that it needs to perform at the most optimal level of functioning.

When engaging in yoga breathing, the body brings in extra supplies of air that cause the blood stream to be purified and rejuvenated with more oxygen. Since oxygen is proven to recharge the body's batteries in a number of ways, saturating the blood with extra levels of the nutrient dramatically increases the energy flowing through our bodies.

Researchers have discovered that oxygen is the most critical chemical ingredient for the body's production of Adenosine Triphosphate

(ATP), which is our main source of energy. Despite popular belief that most of our energy is taken in through the foods we eat, respiration delivers the highest quantity of energy that is needed to keep us thriving with vitality.

If done properly, deep yoga breathing can help individuals stave off a number of increasingly prevalent disorders and diseases. Breathing deeply through the nose decreases the human body's susceptibility to a wide range of bacteria and germs, as the tiny hairs trap the pathogens on their way to our lungs and the immune system gets a boost.

The increased air supply also reduces the risk for developing heart disease or experiencing a stroke because more oxygen is able to improve the circulation of blood and prevent blockages that deprive the heart of its needed nutrients. The Journal of the Royal Society of Medicine also has found that yoga breathing is able to improve adverse symptoms of fatigue, insomnia, anxiety, irritable bowel syndrome, heartburn, constipation, muscle cramping, depression, and vision problems.

In addition to plentiful physical advantages for overall health and well-being, yoga breathing results in a number of exceptional mental benefits. When focusing on breathing, the control shifts from the brain stem, or medulla oblongata to the cerebral cortex of the brain. As various thoughts and emotions are passed, the mind is able to achieve focus and clarity. All forms of emotional stresses, random distractions, and negative thoughts are removed so that prana can freely flow through. Yogis notice considerable boosts in concentration, focus, self-awareness, positivity, inner peace, self-confidence, and acceptance. Focusing so intently on your breathing and the intake of breath into your body has the incredible impact of bringing a unique calmness to the mind and the spirit.

Common Yoga Breathing Exercises

One of the most common breathing exercises in yoga is known as Ujjayi, which translates to mean "victorious breath" in Sanskirt. Ujjayi breathing is beneficial for increasing self-awareness, lowering high blood pressure, reducing rapid heart rate, and removing stress for a more calm and peaceful outlook on your surroundings.

To begin, start with a deep breathing practice in the sitting position with the spine perfectly erect. Then, create a slight hissing sound as you breathe by contracting the back of your throat or epiglottis. Inhale for four seconds through the nostrils while making the Ujjayi sound and exhale for six seconds through the nose with the sound. With practice, the counts and repetitions can be increased. As the breathing stimulates the body's parasympathetic nervous system, it has the profound effect of inducing relaxation of both the body and mind.

Another yoga breathing exercise that can be practiced by both beginners and advanced yogis alike is called Surya Bhedan, which translates to mean "revitalizing breath" in Sanskirt. Since the practice involves breathing through the right nostril, it has been associated with increasing prana, revitalizing the physical energy of the body, boosting the efficiency of the digestive tract, and augmenting the sympathetic nervous system.

Beginners should start with a deep breathing practice before using the right hand to close the left nostril. Without strain or force, inhale through the right nostril for four seconds and exhale for six seconds. Practicing this breathing exercise for just five minutes can help remove the Kafa imbalance and increase body temperature to benefit with weight loss.

With more people than ever before leading a sedentary life, the world is experiencing a steady climb in the occurrence of modern lifestyle health disorders like heart disease, diabetes, and stroke. This increase can be partly attributed to the fact that almost no human beings are now using the full capacity of their respiratory organs and exercising their lungs for the highest functioning. Luckily, yoga breathing is extremely effective at reversing bad breathing habits to help minimize the risk for these issues.

Although it may take some time to get accustomed to, yoga breathing can eventually reprogram the body's natural breathing processes. Using this guide, retrain your body to make the correct breathing patterns more automatic and you should experience a wealth of health benefits through all aspects of your daily life.

Yoga Seated Postures

This chapter will go over a few of the most common and basic sitting postures for you that anyone can start to implement right away. The seated postures in Yoga are better known as asanas. Asana in Sanskrit simply means sitting. The Yoga sitting postures or asanas are great for helping you get in tune with your mind and body as well as help with flexibility.

These asanas are ideal to implement when you are practicing breathing exercises, or if you want to start or end your yoga session with meditation. As you get more advanced you will very likely discover that there a significant amount more asanas that you can do, but for the purposes of this book I will just show a few basic's for beginners. You very well may not even have a need or desire to go beyond these postures as well, which of course is just fine.

Sukhasana: The Easy Posture

This is the first posture that is highly recommended for beginners to try because…well just like the name implies it is pretty easy. Not only is it easy to do but it also helps increase your flexibility in your hips and spine which will help with more challenging yoga poses. The instructions are as follows:

1. Sit cross-legged on the floor with each foot underneath the opposite knee.
2. Sit up straight with your head looking forward and lengthen your spine by slightly arching back and sticking out your chest with your shoulders slightly back.
3. Put your hands on your knees, relax and start to breathing in and out through your nose.

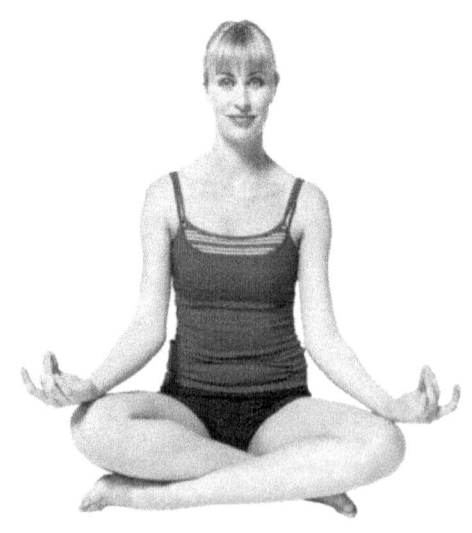

Well that was easy; right? Of course it was. That's why they call it the "Easy Posture." Of course if you don't feel comfortable you can always put cushioning or pillows underneath. That usually should do the trick until your body starts to adjust and become more flexible. Now on to the next one.

Svastikasana: The Auspicious Posture

This posture looks very similar to the previous one except it requires a bit more flexibility. This posture is great for improving the flexibility of the knees, hips and ankles. This posture is also good for strengthening the back as well.

1. Sit with your legs out in front of you. Take hold of one foot and place it along the inside of the opposite thigh.
2. Then bend your knee so you can grab your other foot with both hands and slowly put between your thigh and calf
3. With palms on both knees, lengthen your spine by keeping erect and slightly stretch it upwards while keeping your head looking forward.

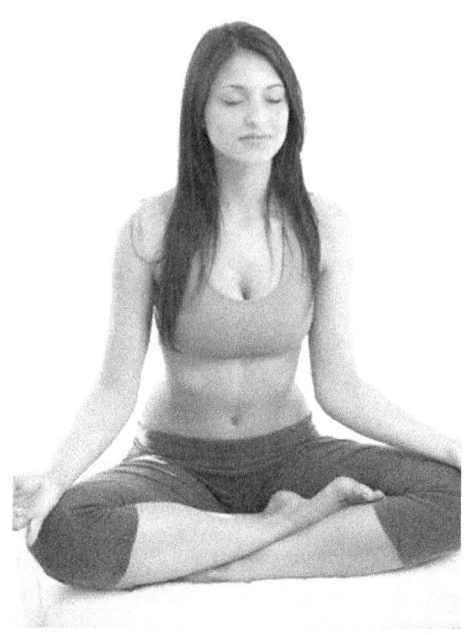

As you can see this posture may look similar but is a bit more difficult. If you feel and pain or discomfort while trying to do this simply stop doing it and revert back to the previous posture mentioned. Once you get more flexible you can then work your way up to this one.

Vajrasana: The Thunderbolt Posture:

Not only is this posture also really easy to implement, but it is also a lot safer for those with back problems as well. Of course you may

want some cushions to put underneath your knees so they don't get
sore.

This posture also helps with flexibility in your thighs and ankles. In
addition, it also known to help with circulation to your abdomen and
improving digestion. Awesome right? Well here is how you do it.

1. Kneel on the floor and sit back on your heels. Rest your hands
   on your knees.
2. Stretch your spine upwards to lengthen your spine and look
   forward.

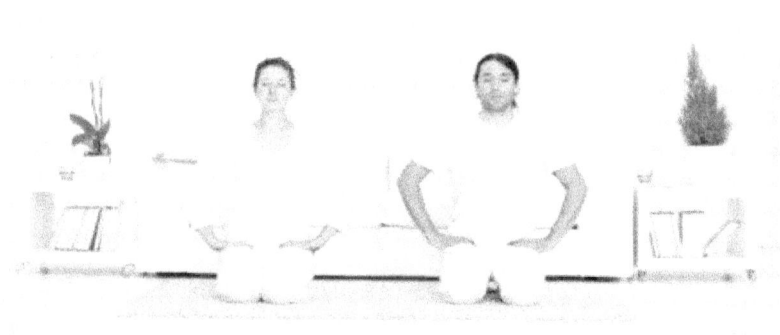

There you go. It's that simple. Now to the final sitting pose.

Balasana: Child Pose

This is not a traditional sitting posture but it is a pose that you will very likely find yourself in during yoga and it is a great pose to meditate or reflect and since you are on your knees on the ground I included it in this section. You will find this position easy and very relaxing and certainly can be used solely for meditative purposes.

1. While on your knees, lower your hips to your heels.

2. Then move forward placing your forehead to the floor and
    stretch your arms out in front of you with your palms on the
    floor.

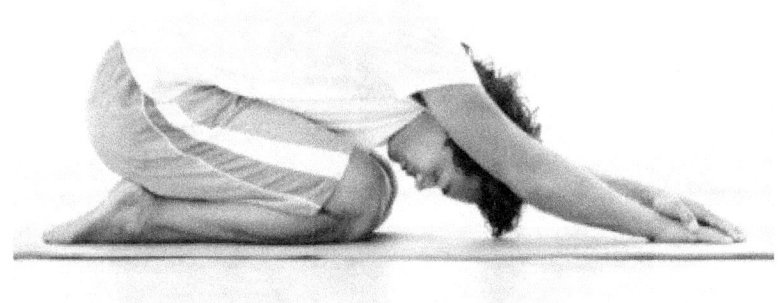

There you have it. As you can see there is not much to these poses at
all, yet they are a very important component to yoga. As mentioned
before not only are they great for meditating but they can increase your
flexibility to help you with more advance postures, including most
standing postures which I will go into next.

Yoga Standing Postures:

What really separates yoga apart from most meditation practices are the standing postures along with the twisting postures as well. While the seated postures are more for preparation and meditative purposes, the standing postures is where you will actually start practicing yoga.

Standing is one of the most basic physical human behaviors that we do on a daily basis and often do not contemplate in the least. However, if you have ever tripped, slipped, or taken a tumble, you may be more conscious of the importance of balance in standing.

It is essential that individuals develop a strong centered equilibrium of inner and outer core strength to stand up tall and gain stable upright balance. As a result, various forms of yoga have placed an emphasis on learning and practicing standing postures to develop greater strength, balance, flexibility, and stamina.

Similar to the seating postures, there are so many different standing postures possibly even more so that I certainly will not cover them all in this book. Therefore since I assume that you are a beginner, I am just going to be going over the most common basics which will be more than enough to get you started with practicing yoga.

Whether you just want to learn the basics to moderately improve your health or flexibility, or you want to evolve and become more advanced, these positions are essential for you to know. As you will eventually learn you will notice that many of the advanced postures derive from the more basic postures. So here are some of the standing postures that you can start working on right away and start acquiring some experience with practicing yoga.

Tadasana: Mountain Posture

This is the most simple and basic posture that there is in yoga. In most yoga classes or routines you will very often find yourself starting in this standing position. Many of the other yoga standing positions are derived or transitioned from this position so it only makes sense to start out with this one. It is also very easy for anyone to do.

1. Stand straight up with your feet either about hip width apart or close together. Make sure at least your heals are not touching. Simply relax and with your arms to your sides looking straight ahead.

2. Take several deep breaths in and out preferably through
    your nostrils.

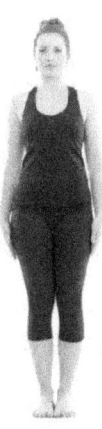

Well that about sums it up for this one. As you can see this is one that
anyone should be able to do. But don't worry. It will get a little bit
more challenging from here. Now to the next one.

Uttanasana: Forward Bend

When beginners and advanced yogis alike practice the Forward Bend, there are numerous therapeutic and revitalizing benefits. Since the head is below the heart in this standing posture, it allows the blood to slowly rush towards the head and give brain cells an invigorating boost of oxygen.

In addition to keeping the spine very strong and flexible, the pose is efficient at reducing depression levels, providing energy to fight chronic fatigue, calming the mind, activating the core muscles, easing headaches and asthma symptoms, stimulating the kidneys, enhancing digestion to combat constipation, and lowering high blood pressure.

1. Beginning in a standard Mountain Pose with your hands on your hips, inhale and bring your arms up over your head.
2. Then exhale and fold forward from your hips. Make sure that you lengthen your abdomen as much as possible as you move fully into the deep bended position.
3. While keeping your knees and thighs straight, place your fingertips on the floor beside your feet or hold the back of your ankles with your palms. If needed, it is possible to modify the pose by crossing your forearms and holding your elbows.

4. Lengthen the front of your torso with each inhalation and release more deeply into the folded Forward Bend pose with every exhalation. Allow your head to hang freely from the base of your neck and release all of the tension that tends to build up between the shoulder blades.

5. After staying in the pose anywhere from 5 to 6 breaths, bring your hands to your hips and slowly start to roll up to exit the pose and reaffirm the lengthening of the abdomen.

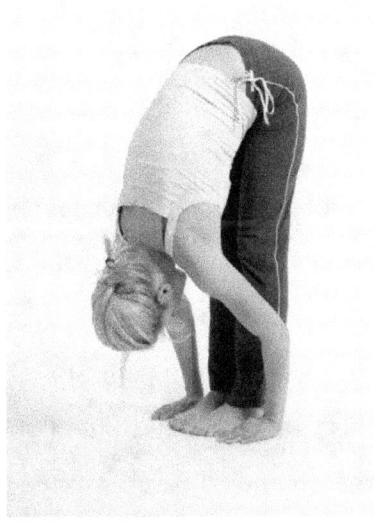

Ardha Uttanasana: Half-Forward Bend

The Half-Forward Bend is highly effective at stretching your hips, thighs, knees, hamstrings, calves, abdominals, and lower back for a strengthening of your muscles. Since the pose is excellent for warming up the body and engaging the core, it is often used as preparation for other kinds of forward bends in yoga practices.

Beyond the physical benefits for improving posture, this pose also helps beginners learn how to link their breathing with movement, which in turn soothes and calms the mind to relieve anxiety or stress.

1. Starting in the mountain pose inhale and bring your arms up over your head like in the   regular forward bend.

2. Exhale and bend forward from your hips. Then inhale and extend your arms straight out in front of you and bend your knees. Your arms should be parallel to the floor. You can either look either slightly down or straight ahead just as long as head in neutral position between your arms.

3. Hold for 5 to 6 breaths then come back up and repeat as desired.

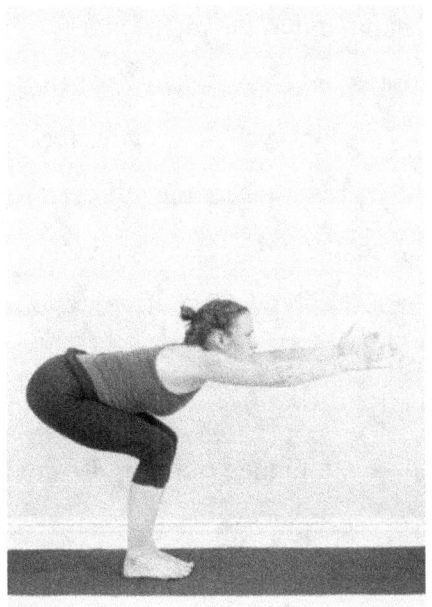

Utthita Trikonasana: Triangle Pose

Through the total expansion of your chest and shoulders in Triangle Pose, you will notice that you have increased mobility within your hip joints and neck. The posture truly stretches a multitude of muscles in your spine, thighs, calves, hamstrings, and hips for toning.

This standing posture also has been linked to relieving stress, improving digestion, alleviating symptoms of menopause, enhancing fertility, and stimulating the increased function of all abdominal organs.

1. Begin by standing tall at the top of your yoga mat in Mountain
   Pose and taking a large step backwards with your right foot
   about three feet behind you. Turn your foot pointing towards
   the side of the mat while keeping your left foot pointing
   forward. As you inhale deeply, reach both of your arms out to
   form a "T-shape" with your shoulders relaxed and your palms
   pointing down.

2. Now, exhale as you hinge your hips downward towards your
   left leg so that your hipbone meets your pelvis. Keeping the
   spine elongated, continue to reach your right arm over the top
   of your head towards the sky. Enable your left hand to float
   towards your left shin and lift your knee cap on your front
   thigh.

3. In order to support your lower spine, be sure to draw in your
   lower abdomen and tuck your chin in slightly to lengthen the
   top of your neck. Turn the back foot just slightly to limit the
   force being placed on the Sacroiliac joint to minimize the risk
   of creating lower back pain. Inhale and exhale comfortably
   while holding the position to maintain a strong connection with
   the earth.

4. On an exhale, exit the pose by looking down towards your left
    foot, pulling your lower abdomen in, rooting down through
    your feet, and inhaling as you rise back up into a standing
    position. Repeat on the other side.

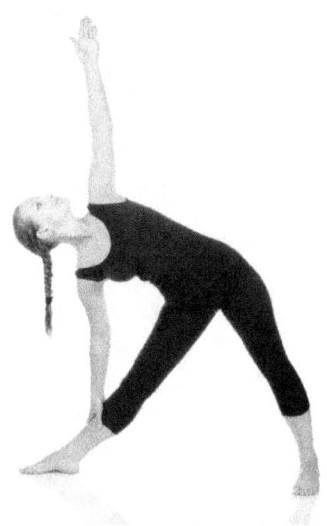

Virabhadrasana I: Warrior I

As its name suggests, the Warrior I posture aims to release
practitioners' inner spiritual warrior who can bravely fight against the
universal enemy of self-ignorance that leads to all of human suffering.
This standing posture is highly effective at strengthening the muscles
of the back, toning abdominal muscles for a stronger core and
improved digestion, relieving the pain of sciatica, and strengthening
the hips. It has also been proven to help yogis develop stamina,

endurance, balance, focus, concentration, and self-awareness at the core.

1. Standing in Mountain Pose, take a deep exhalation and step your right foot forward about 3 feet. Your left leg should be straight. Arms should be dangling along your side.

2. Inhale and raise your arms up over your head and bend your right knee at a 90 degree angle so that your thigh is parallel to the floor.

3. Hold this position for 3 to 4 breaths.

4. On your last exhale straighten out your right leg and bring your arms back down to their original position.

5. Come back to Tadasana and repeat on opposite side.

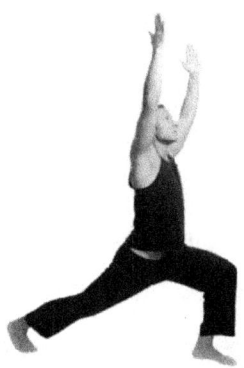

Virabhadrasana II: Warrior II

As a powerful stretch for the legs, chest, and groin muscles, the deep hip-opening Warrior II pose helps to tone the muscles of the thighs, buttocks, abdomen, ankles, and even the arches in the feet. Since the movement opens the chest, it has been linked to improving breathing capacity, relieving symptoms of asthma, and enhancing the circulation of blood to the heart.

For pregnant women, Warrior II is especially helpful for increasing energy, relieving chronic backaches, and stimulating healthy digestion. Like a warrior, yogis who practice this standing posture regularly notice a clearer mind with stronger abilities to concentrate without distraction.

1. For this variation of the Warrior pose, start by walking your feet about four feet apart or as wide as you are able to comfortably stretch.

2. As you inhale raise your arms to be parallel with the floor, reach your arms actively out at the sides, spread your shoulder blades wide, and face your palms downwards.

3. Turn your right foot slightly to the right while positioning your left foot at a 90 degree angle, but ensure that both heels are properly in line. As you exhale start to turn your left thigh outwards so that the left knee is aligned with the left ankle. Keep your pose grounded by strengthening the right leg and firmly pressing the right heel into the floor

4. Using your middle finger as a focal point, turn your gaze forward over your left arm and breathe calmly. After 4 to 6 breaths or as much as you desire, on an inhale straighten your right leg and exhale while you start to lower your arms to your sides. Repeat process on opposite side.

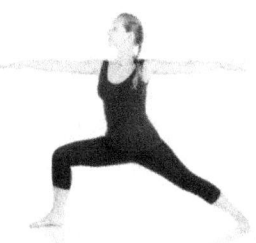

Adho Mukha Svanasana: Downward-Facing Dog

Although Downward-Facing Dog is one of the common poses within the traditional Sun Salutation sequence, it can be an excellent yoga asana individually to reap countless health benefits. As a mild inversion standing posture, it is able to effectively calm the human central nervous system to relieve symptoms of stress, anxiety, insomnia, asthma, high blood pressure, sinusitis, and mild depression. By calming the mind and energizing the body with a strong stretch of various muscles, the Downard-Facing Dog has been proven to alleviate symptoms or discomfort associated with both menstruation and menopause.

1. Beginning on the floor positioned on your hands and knees, place your knees directly below your hips and your hands slightly forward of your shoulders. Straighten your arms and inhale.

2. On an exhale, lift your knees off the floor and lengthen your legs without locking your knees and stick your buttocks up in the air. Your ears should be right between your arms.

3. Stretch your heels down towards the floor, but make sure you do not lock your straightened knees. If you can't put your heels on the floor then do the best you can do. Your head should be pressed toward your feet. Emphasize the lengthening in your spine as you equally distribute your weight onto your hands and feet.

4. Hold this standing posture for 5 to 6 slow breaths or as long as desired. When exiting the pose on an exhale, bend your knees back to the floor and rest in Child's Pose for several breaths.

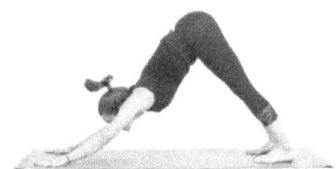

And just for fun, since it is called the Downward Dog pose I thought it would be somewhat appropriate and even humorous to include a dog

performing the pose. It's actually doing a pretty decent job, but I
advise you to emulate the first picture ☺

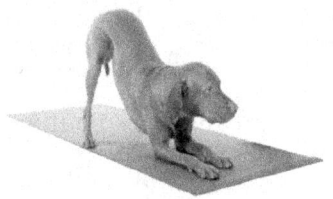

Vrikshasana: Tree Pose

Here is a more challenging pose for you. As the ultimate standing
posture for improving your sense of balance, the Tree Pose is
extremely beneficial for strengthening the muscles in your inner
thighs, calves, ankles, hips, groins, spine, feet, and shoulders.

This Tree Pose has been proven to be effective at increasing mind and
body awareness, calming the central nervous system, relaxing the
mind from stress, enhancing posture, relieving sciatica pain, reducing
flat feet, and building self-esteem.

1. While standing in the Mountain Pose inhale and begin by shifting your weight slightly onto your left foot and keeping it firmly pressed into the floor for support.

2. Exhale as you bend your right knee, reach down with your right hand to clasp your right ankle and draw it up against your inner left thigh. If possible without strain, press your right heel into your left groin with your toes pointing downwards towards the floor. Make sure that your pelvis is centered directly over your left foot for optimal balance.

3. Now lengthen your tailbone towards the floor and firmly press your right sole against your left thigh. If you are not that flexible you can place your foot on your ankle. As you inhale raise your hands upwards towards the ceiling. If you want you can put your arms together like in the picture below or just have them straight up. If you struggle with balance you can also have your arms straight out at your sides as well.

4. Gaze steadily at a chosen fixed point in front of you. After holding the posture for 4 to 6 breaths or as long as you desire, release your right leg, step back into Mountain Pose and exhale. Repeat on the opposite leg.

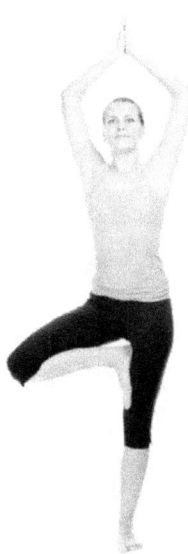

Although these standing postures will take time for patience and practice, always remember to breathe smoothly, focus your gaze, keep a calm mind, and come into the poses slowly. Standing postures are an excellent method for beginners to learn how to be more aware of how to position various parts of your body, including your legs, arms, head, trunk, chest, and feet.

After mastering the basic elements of alignment within the foundation of standing postures, it will become easier to turn the awareness inward to bring about a steadiness of both body and mind in other seated or bended yoga poses. More than being able to stand steadily on one foot, improved balance will ensure you find true physical, emotional, and mental stability.

Yoga Bending Postures:

In yoga the body part that is considered to be the center of focus is your spine. Your spine is known as the central channel for energy and consciousness. The energy is said to flow through your spine to the top of your head bringing you a supreme level of consciousness. Therefore in practicing yoga it is important to focus on strengthening your spine and making it more flexible, which is the intent of these postures.

If you find yourself hurting when doing these than simply ease up and do the best that you can do without causing pain or discomfort. As time goes on you will eventually get better at them. This section is going to cover some of the most basic and common twisting or bending postures in yoga. Of course this isn't anywhere near all of them, but these are the ones that are most suitable for beginners to try out. So with that let's go into our first bending posture.

Bhujangasana: Cobra

The cobra is focused on lying face down and opening your chest which can increase your lung capacity. This also really focuses on the upper back and also increases flexibility in your arms, chest and shoulders. It also isn't too difficult to do as you will see.

1. Lie face down on the floor with your legs spread at hip width. Bend your elbows and place your hands on the floor with you palms down in front of you. Make sure you are relaxed. (To make it easier on your back you can either place your forearms down, or have your hands further out. In addition to make it more challenging you can try to have your arms straight out with your palms together not touching the ground at all.)

2. Inhale as you use your hands to push off the floor by raising your head and chest. Look straight forward and stay relaxed. Make sure your pelvis and ribs stay on the ground.

3. Stay in this position for a few seconds than slowly lower your head back to the floor as you exhale.

4. Repeat several times with the last time taking several breaths in and out while you are facing up before you go back down.

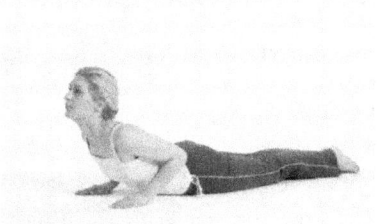

Please note that if you feel like you can do it, you can raise your chest up a little higher if you like. Otherwise doing it like in the picture above is just fine.

Upward Facing Dog:

You will most likely find that this pose is very similar to the previous Cobra pose and it is. However there are a couple of key differences. This pose you are using your arms and hands to absorb the stretch instead of your chest. Therefore your arms will be right underneath your shoulders straightened out. Also you would want to slightly lift your pelvis and abdomen.

Here are the steps for this pose.

1. Start out on your hands and knees looking forward.

2. Start to lower your hips to the floor and pushing off your palms push your shoulders back and up and have your chest out and look up.

3. Inhale and if you can lift your thighs off the floor. Otherwise the pelvis and abdomen are fine. Breathe in and out 3 to 4 times. With your last breath, inhale and as you exhale slowly bring yourself back to your hands and knees. Repeat as much as you want.

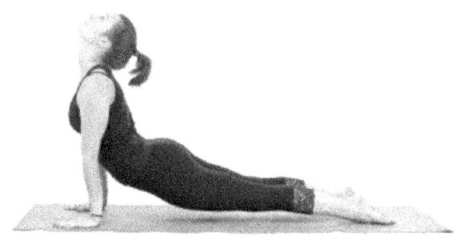

Seated Side Bend:

This is great for increasing flexibility in your rib cage and abdomen as well as your spine. Remember to not hurt yourself by overextending. Do the best you can do and progress gradually.

1. Sit in a cross-legged position or whatever seated position is comfortable to you. Place your left forearm on the floor near your left hip. (If you can't quite reach your left forearm to the ground you can just use your left palm.)

2. Inhale and raise your right arm out to your side and over your head.

3. Exhale while you place your left forearm or palm further out to your left letting your side and right arm bend over to your left side. Inhale and bring yourself to the upright position and repeat 3 – 4 times with the final time breathing in and out several times while extended before you bring yourself back to regular position.

4. Repeat exact sequences on opposite side.

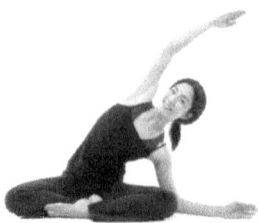

Janushirshasana: Head to Knee

This is a simple pose that stretches your back. It is actually a pretty common stretch so you may have seen it before. Not only is it good for flexibility but also is known to activate your central channel which is as explained earlier you're the pathway to supreme consciousness.

1. Sit on the ground with your legs stretched out and bring your left foot to your right inner thigh.

2. With your spine straightened, inhale and bring your arms up straight up and extended over your head.

3. While you exhale proceed to bend forward bringing your head and chest towards your right leg. Hands can be on the floor or if you can reach out to your foot or toes.

4. Hold for 3 to 4 breaths then come back up with your arms back up over your head. Repeat three to four times or as much as desired.

5. Repeat on opposite side.

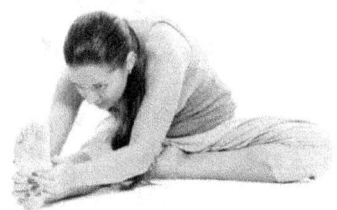

Sitting Twist:

Here is a simple twist to help you with your spine. It can

1. Sit cross-legged with spine straight up or you if you prefer you can sit on a chair or exercise ball like in the picture below.
2. Put your left hand on your right knee and place your right hand right behind you and start to inhale.
3. Start to exhale while twisting head and torso to your right.
4. Hold for a few breaths, then go back to original position. Repeat 3 to 4 times or as much as you want.

5. Repeat on opposite side.

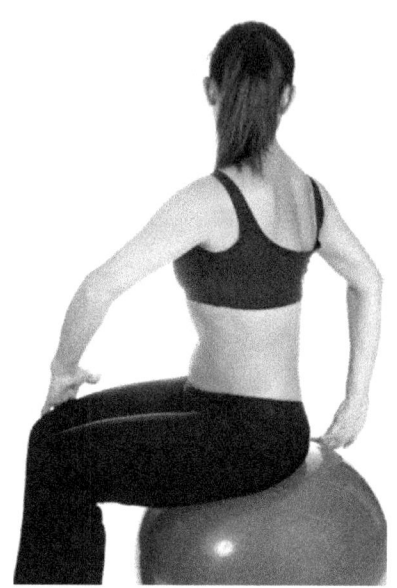

Sage Twist:

This is a slightly more complicated sitting twist but if you can do it you can get a slightly better stretch for your spine.

1. Sit on the floor with your legs out extended in front of you. Bring up your left knee with your left foot right next to your right thigh.

2. Put your left hand on the floor behind you and wrap your right hand around your knee and inhale as you lift your spine straight up.

3. Exhale and twist your head and torso to your left and hold for a few breaths before you come back looking forward. Repeat 3 to 4 times or as much as you want.

4. Repeat on opposite side

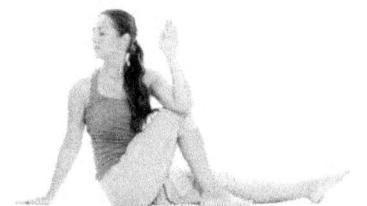

Cat-Cow Pose:

Here is a good pose to help ease your back and neck tension.

1. While on your hands and knees with your back flat take a deep breath in.

2. On the exhale, round your spine up by pushing your belly button up towards the spine. Put your chin down towards your chest. This should resemble a cat to an extent.

3. Inhale and lower your belly back down while arching your upper back and tail bone. Your head should be facing slightly up. This is the cow aspect of the pose.

4. Then on the inhale push your belly button back up and lower your tail bone and head again tucking your chin towards your chest. Repeat this for 30 seconds to a minute or for however long you desire.

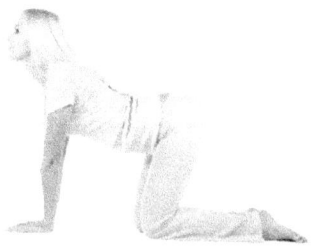

And of course just for fun. This what you will try to resemble ☺

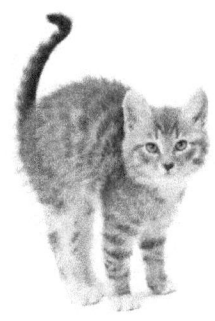

Ardha Virabhadrasana I: Low Warrior I Pose

Here is a stretch modification of the Warrior I pose. This is great for stretching and toning your body particularly the shoulders and hips.

1. On your hands and knees, place your left knee between your hands.

2. With you back leg on the floor, place your hands your left knee. Draw your shoulder blades back to open up your chest.

3. Inhale and bring your arms slowly up. You can either have the straight up or palms together. If you can try to arch back for a deeper stretch. Hold for several breaths.

4. On an exhale, bring your arms slowly back down and go back to your hands and knees.

5. Repeat on opposite side.

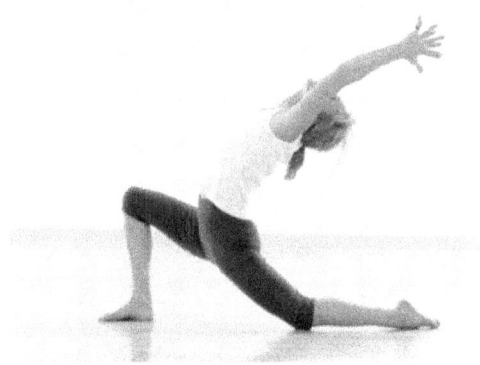

Sample Beginner Routine

Now that I explained some of the common postures in yoga you may want an idea on how they can all flow together. So in this section I decided to show you a good sample yoga routine for beginners that you can start to implement today.

Tadasana (Mountain Pose)

1. Begin by simply standing with your legs together, your big toes touching, and your heels slightly apart so that your second toes are parallel to one another. Lift the balls of your feet and spread your toes before lying them softly back onto the floor.

2. With your weight evenly balanced on your feet in an upright stance, firm your thigh muscles and lift your inner ankles to strengthen the arches of your feet. Imagine a line of energy flowing along your inner thighs to your groins and through the core of your torso to the top of your head.

3. Pressing your shoulder blades into your back, widen your shoulders and then release them down your back. Without

pushing your ribs forward, lift your sternum straight towards the sky and widen your collarbones for a strong posture.

4. Now with your arms to your sides lift up your right arm straight forward and overhead and turn your head to the left and inhale. Hold for a couple seconds and bring your arm back down and your head forward. Exhale. Repeat with bringing your left arm up while inhaling and turning your head to the right. Exhale as you come back to normal position. Repeat this sequence 8 -10 times.

5. Remain in mountain pose and concentrate on your breathing. This is pretty much just a warm up which is essential for the rest of this beginner yoga routine. Breathe slowly and fluidly as your hold the Mountain Pose from 30 seconds to one minute.

Virabhadrasana I (Warrior I Pose)

1. From Mountain Pose, step or lightly jump your feet apart on an exhale so that they are separated by three or four feet apart. Lift your arms to be perpendicular to the floor and parallel to one another while reaching actively through your fingers towards the ceiling

2. Next, turn your left and right foot towards the right. While aligning both of your heels, rotate your torso on an exhale to the right. As you continue to breathe without strain, exhale and

bend your right knee to be positioned directly over the right ankle with your shin perpendicular to the floor.

3. Lift your ribcage away from your pelvis as you strongly reach upwards with your arms. Feel the energy running up the back of your leg, across your abdomen and chest, and up into your arms as you raise them high. If comfortably possible, bring the palms together and spread the palms against each other to reach higher.

4. Hold the Warrior I Pose anywhere from 30 seconds to one minute while breathing slowly. To exit, lower your arms and place your hands back onto your hips on an exhale. Inhale as your firmly press into your right heel and step your left leg forward. Adjust your feet back to Mountain Pose, repeat the motion on the opposite left side, and return to Tadasana.

Virabhadrasana II (Warrior II Pose)

1. 1. After standing back in Mountain Pose, begin the next pose by stepping or lightly jumping your feet to be three or four feet apart. Raise your arms to be parallel with the floor and reach them out to the sides with your shoulder blades spread wide. Turn your right foot slightly towards the right and your left foot out to the left at a 90-degree angle with both heels aligned.

2.   From the space between your shoulder blades, stretch your arms away and keep them parallel to the floor without leaning your torso. Ensure that both sides of your abdomen are equally long and that your shoulders are positioned directly over your pelvis bone. Slightly turn your head towards the left to gaze out over your arm towards your fingers.

3.   As you aim your focus and concentrate on slow deep breaths, hold the pose for 30 seconds to one minute. Exit the pose on an inhale to come back to Mountain Pose. Then, switch sides to repeat the steps on the left for the exact same length of time before returning to Mountain Pose in preparation for the next pose.

Uttihita Chaturanga Dandasana (Plank Pose)

1.   From Mountain Pose, move onto your hands and knees on your yoga mat. Bring your palms directly under your shoulders and spread the fingers wide with each middle finger pointing forward.

2.   Now, step one foot back and then the other so that your legs are straight with your toes tucked underneath. Engaging the core muscles in the abdominals, press out through your heels and firm your legs to hold the Plank Pose. If at all possible, your body should be one straight line without sagging or arching any part.

3. While pressing your front thighs towards the ceiling, firm your
    shoulder blades against your back to spread them away from
    the spine. Imagine pushing the floor away from you so that
    there is as much space as possible between the ground and your
    chest for the ultimate stretch.

4. Hold this pose for anywhere from 30 seconds to one minute.
    Then, exit the pose by gently releasing your legs to bring your
    knees back down to the mat. Rest on your knees for a few
    seconds before moving into the next pose.

Urdhva Mukha Svanasana (Upward-Facing Dog)

1. After kneeling, move into a prone position lying on the floor by
    rolling forward over the toes and stretching your legs back.
    Bend your elbows and spread your palms on the floor beside
    your waist to keep your forearms perpendicular to the floor.

2. Inhale gently as your press your inner hands firmly into the
    floor and straighten your arms. Lift your torso up towards the
    ceiling and your legs a few inches off the floor. Be sure to
    narrow the hip points and firm the buttocks to lift the pubic
    bone towards the belly button.

3. Although it is important to not push the ribs forward, lift
    through the top of your sternum and firm your shoulder blades

against your back. Gaze straight ahead or slightly tip your head back without compressing the back of the neck.

4. While breathing easily and naturally, hold the pose anywhere from 15 to 30 seconds. Gently release to the floor and move back onto your hands and knees to position for the Cat-Cow Pose.

Maryjaryasana Bitilasana (Cat-Cow Pose)

1. Lift back onto your hands and knees in a tabletop position with your wrists aligned directly beneath your shoulders and your knees positioned in line with your hips. Make sure your elbows and shoulders are also aligned perpendicular to the floor underneath your hands.

2. As you inhale your next breath, lift your buttocks and chest towards the ceiling. While your belly gently drops towards the floor, lift your head to gaze straight forward. If you are having difficulty reaching the full stretch, it is recommended that you curl your toes under.

3. On a deep exhale, pull your spine towards the ceiling to round out your back and allow your head to slightly drop down. Focusing on your navel, ensure the tops of your feet lay flat against the floor.

4. Come back into the Cow Pose on an inhale and then exhale as you return to the rounded back positioning of Cat Pose. Repeat this sequence for 10 to 20 times for a gentle flowing vinyasa. Then, give yourself a chance to rest by sitting back on your heels and breathing soothingly in preparation for the next pose.

Adho Mukha Svanasana (Downward-Facing Dog)

1. Begin by moving back onto your hands and knees just like the previous Cat-Cow Pose, with your knees directly below your hips and hands slightly forward of your shoulders. Spread your palms outwards so that your index fingers are parallel or slightly turned to out towards the mat.

2. As you exhale, lift your knees away from the floor and push your hips towards the sky. At first, keep your knees just slightly bent and heels lifted off the floor to accommodate the stretch. Gently against the natural resistance, lift your buttocks upwards. On another exhalation, push the top of your thighs back so that your heels can stretch back onto the floor and your body attains an inverted "V" shape.

3. Once your legs are straight, firm your outer arms and actively press the base of your index fingers into the floor. Keeping your head positions between your upper arms without letting it

hang freely, continue working on your yoga breathing exercises to calm your mind.

4. Remain in this Downward-Facing Dog Pose anywhere from one to three minutes, depending on your level of comfort. Then, exit the pose by bending your knees back onto to the floor with an exhalation for rest.

Balasana (Child's Pose)

1. Begin the final resting pose by kneeling on the floor and sitting on your heels with both big toes touching together. Then, separate your knees to be aligned at the same width as your hips. On an exhale, lay your torso down between your thighs for a deep forward bend.

2. Now, lay your hands gently on the floor beside your legs with your palms up. Be sure to release the front of your shoulders towards the floor. On each exhale, release tension to get deeper into the flood to lower your chest to your knees as close as comfortably possible without strain.

3. While breathing slowly and gently into your torso, hold this resting pose anywhere from 30 seconds to three minutes. As the pose stretches your hips and lower back, release all of the tension buildup within your body for the ultimate relaxation.

To exit the pose, lengthen the front of your torso and lift up from your tailbone on a final deep calming inhale.

Well there you have it. This is a very good beginner routine to practice. Of course once you get more familiar with this one you can try coming up with your own routines from the poses that you learned from this book. You can either start out with the prior routine and throwing in an extra pose or substituting a pose for another one.

For example after the warrior II pose once you come back to Tadasana you can add in the tree pose. Or you can simply do the tree pose in place of Warrior II. Another thing you can do is from Warrior I you can go right into Warrior II. You would simply turn your torso in a matter so that you are using the same bending knee. So if you have your right knee bent you would turn left and hold your arms out to your sides straight out while you are still bending on your right knee. Then you can go back to Warrior I and then to Tadasana, and then repeat the sequence on the opposite side.

Don't be afraid to have fun and get creative with your routine. Afterall, you don't want to get bored by doing the exact same routine over and over again. Just remember that when you do a routine you typically want to start out with a warm up such as the arm raises or you can simply even do shoulder roll by rolling your shoulders forwards and backwards. Then go ahead with the poses. Make sure that you end with a resting pose such as the Child's Pose or another resting pose.

In fact a great way to end a routine is with what is called Shavasana or the corpse pose. No matter what routine you do it is almost always recommended to perform this pose after every yoga workout. It is one of the more simple poses, but also one of the most effective as least as far as relaxation is concerned. The next section will go into how to perform this relaxing pose.

Shavasana: Corpse Pose

Typically at the end of most yoga sessions is a deep relaxation technique called shavasana or the corpse pose. It is the most simple yoga pose there is. That is because you simply do nothing. You just lie there like a corpse hence, why it is called the corpse pose.

Shavasana will last for a minimum of five minutes and can last for 15 – 20 minutes or even longer if you desire. The longer the duration the better as you will feel that much more relaxed and clear minded. However, just be careful not to go too long as you may get sleepy. Hence this could be a great technique to do right before bed.

How to do Shavasana:

1. The first step in Shavasana is to lie flat on your back with your arms out to your side and palms up.. If you need to place a pillow under your head or any other part of your bode for comfort then go ahead and do so.

2. Focus on your breathing. Then from head to toe, scan each of your body part muscles and picture tension leaving out of each muscle. For instance, start with your eyes, your temple, your mouth, than shoulders and chest to elbows and then your abdomen, and so on until your reach your feet. Focus on one body part at a time for about 5 – 10 seconds before moving to the next.

3. Try now to just completely clear your mind and just let go of every sort of tension and worry. Once your mind is clear for a few seconds imagine your body sinking in the ground and becoming one with the earth. Imagine a nice drizzle of rain coming down on you; the world nurturing you. This tactic will help you relax by becoming one with the earth and temporarily escaping all of your troubles and worries in your life. Another tactic you can try to induce relaxation is to imagine yourself lying on a body of water. With each breath you take moves you down an ocean toward a tropical island paradise. Whatever makes you feel at ease and relaxed would essentially be just fine.

4. Open your eyes. Slowly get up by rolling to your side and use your arms to push yourself up. Stand up and notice how relaxed and clear minded you are.

Final Thoughts:

There you have it. Everything you need to get started in yoga. Of course this definitely should not be your only guide to yoga. This is simply just to get you started with the basics. Down the line you may want to join a yoga class. Nothing compares to receiving tutelage from an instructor in person. If you are doing something wrong the person can come over and correct your posture. You simply can't get that from any book or manual.

If you can't afford to take any classes right now or don't have the time, the next best thing is to try out a yoga dvd. They obviously cannot analyze you in person, but you can at least see the poses being done in action with the instructor explaining exactly what you should be doing.

Whatever route you decide to go from here doesn't really matter just as long as you keep practicing. Don't worry about whether or not you are doing the poses perfectly, or if you'll look bad in class compared to the other students. Remember we all had to start from somewhere.

Not to mention that yoga is not about perfection. It is simply about doing and improving. You don't have to necessarily have the poses down perfectly to benefit from yoga. Remember that reaching the full benefits of yoga is a marathon not a sprint. It is not something you achieve within a few months, but rather a lifetime endeavor. You can say it is even a change in lifestyle. So as long as you commit from here going forward that you are going to practice on an almost daily basis, then you are well on your way to reaping the full benefits of yoga. And with that I wish you well on your yogic journey.

Please Leave Review:

I sincerely hoped you found this book an enjoyable read and helpful as well. If you could be so kind to leave me a review I would greatly appreciate it. This way I know if I am meeting consumer's expectations and if there is anything I can improve on. Thank you.

Other Books by Max Fischwell:

Meditation 101: How Anyone Can Easily
Learn to Meditate Even if You Can't Sit Still:

Free Yourself From the Shackles of Clutter:

Free Yourself From the Shackles of Negative
Thinking:

www.ingramcontent.com/pod-product-compliance
Lightning Source LLC
Chambersburg PA
CBHW060154290526
45789CB00003B/1041